HOW TO BOOST
METABOLISM

How To Boost Metabolism

Increase Metabolism For A Quick Weight Loss

Simon Bareilles

Table of Content

Weight Loss Through Better Metabolism

Those who have heard about metabolism would know it's relation to weight loss. However, there is more to metabolism than weight loss. It is also about how to be healthier. In this book, although we understand that you desire to lose weight, by looking to boosting your metabolism, you will be able to maintain your weight in the long term.

Throughout this book, you would learn the importance of metabolism. You would learn about how you could fire up your metabolism.

If you have tried to boost up your metabolism in the past but didn't achieve any substantial results, you have got the right book to help you with it.

This book would do exactly that - help you with understanding metabolism and knowing how to boost it. Let's get started!

Chapter One: Basics of Metabolism

About Metabolism

In the most basic understanding of metabolism, it is simply how the body converts calories from the food you eat into energy. Metabolism is a series of chemical reactions which gives your body energy to do what it needs to ensure it is functioning. Needless to say, it also keeps you living.

If you don't have metabolism, you wouldn't be able to move of think properly. Metabolism provides the energy for your body and your individual organs to work smoothly.

Consider this; if your heart stops beating, you will invariably die. It is similar to metabolism. If your metabolism stops you wouldn't have the energy for your heart to beat or even breathe!

How Does Your Metabolism Functions

To understand how your metabolism functions, it is important to first understand how you chew and swallow your food. When you eat your food, you will chew and swallow your food. Your food would go down to your digestive tract.

Digestive enzymes break down the food. Fatty food would be turned into fatty acids.

Carbohydrates to glucose and protein into amino acids.

After the food has been broken down, they would be absorbed by the bloodstream and subsequently carried over to the cells. Other hormones and enzymes would then work to convert these nutrients into cells in the body or building blocks for tissues. It may even release them to supply the body as energy supply.

Different Metabolism Components

The two basic metabolic processes are constructive and destructive.

The constructive metabolic process is responsible for building and keeping energy for your body's use. This process is called anabolism.

The destructive is responsible for breaking down nutrients molecules to release energy for the body. This process is called as catabolism.

The process of anabolism (constructive) helps the growth of new cells, repairing and maintaining of tissues and storing of energy through body fat for future use. Small nutrient molecules are converted into larger molecules of fat, carbohydrates and protein.

The process of catabolism (destructive) is responsible for providing immediate energy for the body to use. Instead of building up (anabolism process), this process would break down the nutrient molecules to release energy for the body. The two processes doesn't occur at the same time but are balanced in the body.

There are three components in the catabolism process:

1. **Basal Metabolism** - This is often known as resting metabolism, or the metabolism component which keeps you alive by ensuring normal body functions. This basal metabolism is still at work even if you are bedridden. Basal metabolism is your metabolism's main part, as 60-70% of the calories from your food are used for this process. Those who look to lose weight would generally aim for a higher basal metabolic rate (BMR).

2. **Physical Movements** - This ranges from a simple fingers movement to your rigorous exercise. Approximately 25% of

your food intake goes into this component.

3. **Thermic Effect of Food** - This refers to the processing and digestion of the food you partake. About 10% of your food intake are burned through this.

To simplify, the metabolism formula is such:

Basal Metabolism (about 65%) + Physical Movement (about 25%) + Food Digestion (10%) = Calories You Get From Food

Factors Which Affects Your Metabolism

Your metabolic rate, which is an indication of how fast or slow your metabolism works, is influenced by many different factors. This include:

1. **Age** - The younger you are, the faster your metabolism is. Generally speaking, your metabolism would slow down as you age. For men, metabolism declines at 40, while for women, metabolic rate falls as the age of 30.

2. **Gender** - Men have a faster metabolic rate than women because of the larger muscle mass. Muscle

plays an important role in having a fast metabolism.

3.   **Genetics** - I am sure you have seen some people who eat a lot but wouldn't grow fat. This is because of genetics. There are some people who don't eat much but grow fat easily.

4.   **Amount of lean muscle mass** - As like point number 2, when you have more muscle, you generally would have a faster metabolism.

5.   **Diet** - What you eat would help improve your metabolism. Some food help and some food don't. We would discuss this in the further chapters.

6.   **Hormones** - There are some specific hormones which metabolize specific nutrients. Hormones can be affected by several factors. We

would discuss it later. There are some people who have hormonal disorders or imbalances which would affect metabolism severely.

7. **Stress Levels** - Stress is an important factor towards your metabolism. When you are more stressed, the lower your metabolism.

All these factors affect your metabolism is different ways. From here, you would have a rough idea about how to improve your metabolism. But be prepared to put in the effort required.

Before we get into the detailed plan for firing up your metabolism, you need to know the resolve needed to achieve the right metabolism level for you.

Chapter Two: Should You Boost Your Metabolism?

Improving your metabolism isn't only about losing weight. Although everyone seem to think that boosting your metabolism is about weight loss, you have much more to gain by increasing your metabolism. These are among the benefits that you would get when you start increasing your metabolism:

1) **You would lose weight.** This is perhaps the most obvious benefit of boosting your metabolism. When you start increasing your BMR, you would

burn calories much easier when you do your normal daily activities. Even while you are idle, your body would still be performing the daily actions of burning calories. As you increase your metabolism, you could easily shed 3-5 pounds a week. And the best thing is that these changes are long term.

2) **You don't have to worry about eating more.** As you burn calories faster, you could eat more without feeling bad about it. However, this doesn't mean that you should overindulge or snack on unhealthy food mindlessly. You should still eat healthy. The good thing is that you don't have to spend too much time worrying about the quantity of food you eat.

3) **You would look better.** People with faster metabolism would generally have

brighter and more radiant skin. Their faces tend to be pinkish and more alive with color.

4) **You feel more energized.** It is generally been reported that people with faster metabolism feel more energized. Your body would perform more efficiently to release the energy you need to get going.

5) **You will generally feel healthier overall.** As you have a faster metabolism, your body would function more efficiently. From your digestion to your absorption of nutrients, you would feel that all of them have improved. Besides, you wouldn't need to sleep as much as you used too.

Having a great metabolism is perhaps something very helpful to living a quality life. I would guide you on the steps in the further chapter.

Chapter Three:
The Right Mindset

In anything you do, the most important to succeeding is perhaps having the right mindset. When you have the right mindset, you will find that success comes easily to you.

You may wonder why that is so. How does increasing your metabolism have to do with having the right mindset?

The reason is simple; if you have the right mindset, you will know what to expect from the road ahead. Boosting your metabolism is something which isn't easy. If you don't have the right mindset, you will easily give up.

Boosting your metabolism isn't a quick-fix. It is a long term improvement to your life. You don't just put in a few weeks of effort and expect your weight to maintain the same.

The right mindset towards boosting your metabolism is to realize that it is about changing your lifestyle on a whole and the habits associated with it. Though there are some which are considered small changes, you would still be changing the way of life you have become used to. This would be very uncomfortable for most people. Boosting metabolism involves a great deal of discipline and consistency in your actions. If you expect long term results, you would need to make a long term investment towards it.

You need to remember to follow everything that is set in this book. You can't just follow certain advice and ignore some of them. Doing this would see you failing to get the right results. I have done this for hundreds of people to know that if you don't follow everything, you will not succeed.

However, many people would struggle with it. This is because many people lack the motivation to follow through with what they want. For this, I can solve it by asking you to do some visualization.

I want you to start imagining yourself when you start having a higher metabolism. Close your eyes and imagine the dream weight that you always wanted for yourself. How will you feel? When you look at yourself at the mirror, how would you look like?

From here, I would want you to do the same process daily for a few minutes. Then, do the same process for your expectations after three months and six months from here. Note the differences that you see and feel. It is a very good practice to write down your expected outcome. Research has shown that people who write down their goals have a higher chance of reaching them.

This would help you get through the ups and downs of the program. If you are ready for it, I wish you luck. You have just done the most important thing: Knowing what you want from the program. This would be a great help towards reaching your goal of having a higher metabolism.

Chapter Four: Can You Boost Your Metabolism Quickly

As mentioned, you must treat the advice you read in this book as something which you must apply to all components of your life in order to get the best from the program.

First, and perhaps the most important part of boosting your metabolism is exercise. If exercise is done right, it would contribute to raising our BMR. From this book, you would learn the way to exercise smart. When you start exercising smart, and not hard, you would learn how to maintain your motivation to exercise regularly. In this guide, I would share the importance of building the right muscle mass and applying the right exercise intensity.

In the second section, I would discuss about how to eat right. Eating right is not so much about eating less, although many programs advise on it. The way to eat right is to eat smart. From this book, you would learn why is it important to not only consider the food you eat but also how and when you eat.

The final section would be about how you can cope with stress better. I have mentioned about how stress plays an important role in boosting or lowering your metabolism. You should always bear this in mind.

Do take the time to go through all advice given thoroughly. Make sure that they are ingrained in you so you understand the importance of everything that is being mentioned here. Once you start applying the methods, your body would slowly grow.

How To Exercise Smart

There is a big difference between exercising hard and exercising smart. If you are professional athletic, you would definitely need to exercise hard. However, most of us are not and therefore we need to learn to exercise smart instead.

The exercises that I am about to share may be a bit high intensity and may be a bit hard for a few of you. However, you need not do them for long periods. A short burst of those exercises would do more than enough benefits for you. The goal of these exercises is to simply give your metabolism a kick start with an exercise program which takes a short amount of time but gives the greatest results.

The two main elements in the exercise program that I recommend are:-

(1) Strength and resistance training for building lean muscle mass

(2) Interval training for speeding up the metabolic process.

Build Muscle Mass Through Strength And Resistance Training

The exercises in this program are built to help you improve your strength and resistance. To achieve this, considerable tension is applied on the muscles. What you would achieve is an increase in muscle mass in your body.

When you have more muscles in your body, you are better equipped to lose more calories.

Muscles are like fireplace in the body that burn fuel (calories). As you have more fireplaces, you would have more fuel burned. According to a study done, for every pound of muscle that you add to your body, you would burn an extra 40-50 calories a day.

There have been situations where women come to me and say that they worry they would get large muscles like men. However, they need not worry as the women body is distinctly different from men. The muscles women build would not only add an extra dimension to a woman's shape but would also make them look sexier.

While the process of building muscles is usually associated with weight training, this may not always be the case. There are many exercises which don't require weights at all. This is extremely amazing news for those who are on a budget as it means that they wouldn't need any weights at all.

However, it has to be said that having the right equipment would help you achieve your targets much faster. If you are looking to achieve the best results, a combination of exercises which uses equipment and no equipment is required.

We would firstly discuss exercises which involve weight lifting first. Weight lifting is a great muscle building exercise which applies tension to your muscles through carrying weights. The benefits of using weights are that you could easily measure your progress by the number of pounds or grams indicated on each weight. As your body becomes stronger, you could add more weights.

You would need some testing to do if you want to decide how much weight to start off with. The appropriate weight for you would be a weight that puts tension on your muscles but not one which makes you fatigued.

I would heavily recommend doing exercises which could work out several muscles in your body at once. Although it wouldn't be too much a problem if you want to solely focus on a particular muscle, if you are short of time, it's better to focus on exercises that affect various muscles.

Weight Lifting Exercises

Among the various weight lifting exercises you could do include:

1. **Bicep Curl** - This is perhaps the most basic exercises using weights. This exerts

effort on your biceps. To perform this, hold the weights with your palm facing upwards. Bend your elbow to bring the weights to your shoulders. Make sure the weights don't touch your shoulders. Slowly lower it down. Don't straighten the arm.

2. **Bench Press** - This multi-joint exercise works the major muscles of your shoulders, triceps and chest. Lie on a bench and hold the weight over your chest. Do this until the elbow is bent at 90 degrees. Do this until your arms are straighten, the slowly lower back to your starting position.

3. **Concentration Curl** - This exercise works the biceps. On one leg, kneel using the leg opposite the hand you are working with. Hold one weight with your working hand while putting the other hand on your waist. Place the back of the upper arm of your working hand on the inner thigh of

the other leg. You could lean into that leg to raise your elbow a little. Raise the weight in front of your shoulders and then slowly lower the arm until it's almost straight.

4. **Chest Fly** - This works your chest, while emphasizing on your outer muscles. Lie on a comfortable bench while holding onto your weights overhead, palms facing inwards. Lower the weights to your sides up until shoulder level, with your elbow slightly bent. Bring the weights up back to starting position.

5. **Overhead Press** - This exercise works the shoulder muscles. Stand/sit straight. Hold your weights with your elbows bent and your hands in front of your eyes. Bring your weights over the head while keeping your back straight. Gently bring the weights down to starting position.

Exercises Without Weights

To get the best results, strength exercises without weights could be combined with weight lifting exercises for routine. Among them include:

1. **Squat** - The squat is an exercise which works multiple joints including the hamstrings, quadriceps, gluteals and lower back. This is perhaps the one exercise that you must do if you don't plan to use weights. From a standing position, gently lower your body until your knees are bend at a 90-degree angle. Ensure that your feet are flat on the ground. Slowly return to a standing position.

2. **Crunches** - This is one exercise which many people don't do correctly. Although the crunch is well-known for

working out your abs, many people don't do it correctly, and thus won't be able to get the best effect from it. Lie on the floor under a mat with your knees bents and your feet flat on the floor. You may put your hands behind your head.

Gently raise your upper body, until you feel your abs contract. To ensure the tension, don't raise your body to 90 degrees. You could also ensure the tension by not letting your body rest on the floor. Instead, keep yourself slightly elevated from the ground.

3. **Pushups** - This is a very common but effective strength exercise. While the basic pushup works, I recommend adding some complexity to work more muscles.

   You could do pushups in between of two chairs. These also work the chest and triceps. Place both feet on a stable chair and then place both your hands on separate chairs.

The two chairs your hands are resting can have a gap of about 60cm. The chair with your feet should be aligned with the middle of the two other chairs. Your body should also be stretched naturally from the chair at your feet to the chairs in front. Bring your chest down slowly.

When you are planning for strength exercises routine, you would need to understand the various muscle groups to determine which muscles you want to work on. Always remember that multi-joint exercises are better in achieving faster metabolism.

- Deltoids - Caps of your shoulders
- Biceps - Front of your upper arm
- Triceps - Back of your upper arm

- Pectoralis Major - Large, fan-shaped muscle on the front of your upper chest
- Rhomboids - Muscles at the middle of your upper back and between the shoulder blades
- Latisimus Dorsi - Large muscles that go down the middle of your back.
- Lower Back - Erector spine muscles that enables back extension. This muscle is important in maintain strong posture.
- Trapezius - Muscle on your upper back, more commonly known as 'traps'. The upper trap runs from the back of your neck to your shoulder.
- Abdominals - The place where your fat belly goes. The abdomens are composed of external obliques, which trace paths down the sides

and front of the abdomen, as well as the rectus abs - a flat muscle running across the abdomen.

- Quadriceps - Muscles that go up the front of your thighs
- Gluteals - Muscles of your buttocks
- Hamstrings - Muscles located on the back of your thighs
- Hip adductors and abductors - Muscles located on your inner and outer thigh. Abductors on the outside - moving the leg away from your body. Adductors on the inside, pulling your leg to the center of your body.
- Calf - Muscles on the back of your lower leg.

When you have chosen the exercises you want to focus on, you need to think about how intense you want them to be as well as the duration of your exercises. This means the number of repetition and sets.

It largely depends on your tolerance level. Fatigue is a good sign that you have overtaxed yourself. Allow yourself to feel the burn at times but don't push yourself too much.

If you are just starting, always tell yourself to not push yourself too much. Your exercise routine should only last for only 30 minutes or less to gain the optimum results. Also ensure that you shouldn't take more than a 45 second rest between sets to ensure the best results in increasing metabolism.

Strength and resistance exercises are the best way to build muscles for the long term. Don't think about shortcuts like using drugs or steroids to boost growth hormones. While they may improve your performance for the short term, they can have severe long term side effects like liver damage, heart attack and death. Always stick to healthy methods.

People who spend time doing strength exercises have lower blood pressure, improved balance and flexibility. They also have stronger muscles and bones.

Interval training

Interval training is perhaps a method of training that most people fail to understand its importance. Interval training is about having high-intensity exercise and rest. For such training, you need cardiovascular exercise at the highest intensity and then to a lower intensity.

This shift in intensity helps your muscle to adapt to different conditions. This exercise is also called as "metabolic burst" training because this sudden burst in intensity training results in a sudden hike in caloric-losing. Because of this sudden burst, you also suddenly release energy.

Don't underestimate the rest period. The rest periods works as a way for the body to get rid of the waste products in the muscles during the exercise. It's extremely important to keep a moderate intensity during exercise to keep the body in moderate intensity and don't go into total rest. This is to ensure the continuous release of energy.

Interval training is something that could be done for almost any kind of cardiovascular exercise. From running to swimming, this method of training ensures that you build your strength although you are not at your optimum level.

For running, the rest period could be for brisk walking, while for biking and swimming, the activity could be done at a slower but more moderate pace.

Each interval should be around one to four minutes. The resting period could be longer or shorter than your high-intensity exercise, depending on your physical condition. Performing your interval training routine for a total of 30 minutes would already help you achieve optimal results.

Ensure that your moderate intensity exercise really has intensity while allowing your body to rest for the next burst of high intensity exercise. When you start performing during your high intensity exercise, perform your personal best. Being out of breathe is a great sign that you are doing your best.

The best way to determine your highest level of intensity is to calculate your maximum heart rate. To get your maximum heart rate, just subtract your age from 220. A heart rate monitor would be extremely helpful during your exercise as well.

Your pulse rate during moderate intensity exercise should always be greater than your resting heart rate or your normal resting heart rate. To get your resting heart rate, get your pulse rate checked while you aren't exercising.

For those who desire to lose weight, you would expect to lose weight after a few weeks of exercising. Even your normal exercises with moderate intensity will burn more fat than normally.

In a research done, after seven internal workouts over two weeks, the subjects were able to increase their fat burning ability to a staggering 36% just through normal cycling exercises.

After your interval training, you would also develop a "metabolic afterburn". This means that your body would continue to burn calories up to 46 hours after the workout.

Without a doubt, interval training is a more efficient and effective way than cardiovascular training. Normal cardiovascular exercise would also take longer as the objective of it is endurance. This is often goals of marathon runners. However, our goal is not to run marathons but to build metabolism.

Interval training of only 30 minutes or less can deliver significant results in just a couple of weeks.

Develop A Plan

While you choose the specific exercises for your strength and resistance training, coupled with the interval training; you need to have the right schedule to ensure that you are successful. Below is a recommended schedule that you can follow:

Day 1: Strength and resistance exercises

Day 2: Interval training exercises

Day 3: Strength and resistance exercises

Day 4: Interval training exercises

Day 5: Strength and resistance exercises

Day 6: Interval training exercises
Day 7: Rest

From this schedule, it is clear that I recommend an alternate days training schedule. This is intended to facilitate recovery of your muscles. Don't ever perform your strength exercises right after your interval training as this would slow down the muscle building process. I also included a one day rest to ensure that your body makes a full recovery.

You need to make sure that you don't push your body towards fatigue. If you do this, you would trigger a stressful response from your body which severely affects your metabolism. You should also make sure that you breathe normally throughout the exercises so that your body isn't stressed.

I must also stress the importance of warming up before the routine and cooling down after the exercises. Take time to warm up your muscles and breathe deeply as it would help you better in relaxing.

If you feel bored with your routine after some time, change it. Applying variety to your routines may help increase your enjoyment and see which exercises suit you the most.

Other Factors To Consider In Your Exercise Routine

1) **Age Doesn't Matter.** Regardless of your age, you can perform this. For the older people, your interval program may not be as intense at the beginning, but after some time, you could push yourself to increase

the intensity. You may even find yourself pushing yourself more than a younger person.

2) **Exercising More Doesn't Increase Metabolism.** In truth, exercising more only helps you lose weight. But it doesn't help you boost metabolism. Therefore, you shouldn't be too concerned about how much you work out. You should instead be concerned about how intense is your workout. If you feel tired from your workout, take a rest. Don't fatigue yourself. Rest and then go all out on your next workout.

3) **Don't Try Out Other Exercises For The Time Being.** While there are some other exercise routine which may help you, take time to focus on the one I recommend first.

Most exercise program only has a one-time effect. These exercises also guarantee a long-term effect. You would get much more from interval training compared to endurance training as well.

From here, you know the best exercise program to ensure you boost your metabolism. But that's not sufficient. Exercise is only part of your journey towards a faster metabolism. You also need to learn how to eat well.

How To Eat Well

The main fuel for energy lies in your food. Food gives your body the calories needed to burn or store energy. Eating the right food at the right amount and at the right time would result in the best way to improve on your metabolism.

Anyone who is trying to lose weight would need to know that there is a substantial difference between eating to boost your mechanism and eating to lose weight. In traditional dieting, calories are the one you need to look out for.

Many traditional dieting methods put an emphasis on monitoring your calorie intake but the opposite is true for dieting to boost your metabolism. Calories are your friends, if you take the right ones.

When we talk about exercise, I discussed about how building more muscles would ensure that you burn more calories. After you have done interval training for a period of time, your body would burn more calories. To keep up with this calorie burning, you need to eat more.

What Nutrients Are Important

Carbohydrates are perhaps the most important nutrients for firing up your metabolism. At the most basic, they are fuel you use for your daily physical activities. If you are someone who exercises on a regularly basis, carbohydrates are a need. However, if you want to build muscles, there is an added importance to the partaking of carbohydrates.

As you progress in muscle building and interval training, you would need to increase your carbohydrate intake. As your body burns more energy, it would require more energy from carbohydrates.

If you don't take enough carbohydrates, your body turns to your muscle mass for energy. You would have wasted your energy on building weight if you don't consume enough carbohydrates. As a general rule, more than 50 percent of your calorie requirements should come from foods which are rich with carbohydrates.

There are two main types of carbohydrates, simple and complex.

Simple carbohydrates are easier to digest and absorb compared to the complex ones. If you look to build a faster metabolism, you need to focus your diet on taking complex carbohydrates.

Generally, complex carbohydrates are healthy while simple carbohydrates are from processed foods loaded with artificial sweeteners. However, there are also some healthy sources of simple carbohydrates. Examples include fresh fruit juice, milk and honey.

Carbohydrates are not only grains and root crops. There are fibrous carbohydrates as well. This refers to vegetables. Such fiber, although not entirely absorbed by the digestive system, would greatly help the thermic effect. Fiber can help to clean the body as well maintaining its smooth functioning.

Another essential nutrient for faster metabolism is protein. Using amino acids to be processed by the body, the building blocks for cells and muscles is protein. Like complex carbohydrates, protein has a thermic effect as it takes a longer time for the body to break it down.

These are among the healthy sources of protein that you can incorporate into your diet:

1. **Fish** - Fish is a food which has high protein content and is also good for the heart. Cold-water fish like salmon and tuna are especially good for your heart.

2. **Chicken Breasts** - It has the highest amount of protein. Drumsticks are also a good source, but it doesn't have that much of protein compared to the breasts.

3. **Eggs** - Very high in protein. Best thing is that it is cheap too. Eggs contain the important amino acids for growth. The high protein content comes from the egg white and not the egg yolk.

4. **Milk** - Anyone who wants to build muscle need to take milk. Babies are given milk from a tender age because of how important milk is in building up the size of a person.

5. **Whey** - Very high in protein and also very healthy. It is a staple among body builders. It is commonly sold as protein powder.

Contrary to popular belief, fats are an essential part towards building up your metabolism. While too much fat (especially the unhealthy ones) is bad, a bit of healthy fat would help the hormones responsible for metabolism to perform well. Diets which are low or none in fat would lead to bad hormone production and a slower metabolism.

Always focus on the healthy sources of fat like olive oil, avocados, nuts and sunflower seeds.

Calcium is another nutrient which would help you release hormones that boost metabolism. Milk is of course the best source for calcium.

What Nutrients Should You Avoid?

You should always empty calories. This refers to foods which are highly processed and refined. These are normally the simple carbohydrates that aren't natural whole food.

They are empty calories because they fill you up but give little to no nutrients to your body. The worst thing is that such foods would contain a lot of sugar. Examples of food which you shouldn't take include:

- Sweets
- Chocolate Bars
- Chewing Gums
- Pastries
- Cakes
- Soft Drinks
- Fast food

You should also be aware of the effect of caffeine on your body. Too much of it would affect your metabolism terribly. It would trigger a stress response which makes you dependent on it.

What Other Food Should You Take?

- **Soy** - Research has shown that ingesting soy protein would help increase metabolism. However, the soy protein was injected and not fed to subjects. While the research may not be thorough, other research has shown soy to be an incredible food to incorporate into your diet.

- **Spices** - Certain spices like red hot pepper cayenne pepper contain a chemical known as capsaicin which helps raise your metabolism up to 25 percent for around four hours.

- **Green Tea** - If you take green tea on a consistent basis, it will be able to speed up fat oxidation as well as boost metabolism. As green tea also has less caffeine than coffee, it will prove to be a better alternative. Besides, if you don't like the bitter taste of green tea, you can take the capsule ones.

Water To Help Your Metabolism

Drinking eight glasses of water a day is perhaps an advice which is as old as time. This advice also holds true if you are looking to build metabolism as well.

When you are dehydrated, your metabolism would drop. This results in a drop in body temperature. This drop would then trigger your body to store fat to assist your body in increasing or maintaining the body temperature. Besides, when you are active, you would generally need water to maintain your energy levels. If you are someone who sweats a lot , eight glasses of water a day may not even be sufficient. You should drink more than that.

Water plays an important role of cleansing the body of toxins and to enable the body to proceed smoothly with its processes, which includes metabolism.

Time When You Eat

Although you are now consuming the right food, you mustn't neglect the importance of timing when you eat them. This is more important than you can imagine.

Follow these advices to get the best results.

1. **Always Eat Breakfast.** While you are asleep, your body is in starvation mode. To ensure that your metabolism is up

and running, start the day with a hearty and healthy breakfast. You need to remember that the later you have your breakfast, the later your metabolism starts.

2. **Eat Several Meals In A Day.** Ideally speaking, you should look to eat something every two to three hours. If you look to maximize the thermic effect from food, you need to eat more than three meals a day. When you eat every three hours, you would allow the thermic effect to last the entire day. This is because it takes between two and a half to three hours to digest food. Generally speaking, men require 700-1000 more calories each day than women. To break it down, men would require around 6 meals while women need around 5 meals a day.

Don't go over the optimal number of meals and don't do late night snacking. Late night snacking is bad as while you are sleeping; your body can't digest well. It is also recommended to eat foods which are easily digested when you are taking your last meal.

3. **Take A Snack/Meal Right After Your Workouts.** A great hearty meal rich with protein and carbohydrates taken within an hour or so after your workout assists in muscle recovery and building new ones.

4. **Don't Skip Meals.** You should never skip a meal. Even if you have a very busy schedule, make sure that you have food for emergency like biscuits or fruits. It is even recommended to make a shake if you are really rushing for time.

Sample meal plans

I know it is difficult for many of you to decide on what to eat. It can be difficult considering most people are extremely busy nowadays with their own work life and their children.

I have therefore, included two sample meal plans that you can use to assist you. As you can see, both meal plans focus heavily on the combination of protein and carbohydrates. The portions would be decided by you. You would need to decide on the calories you need. Remember that carbohydrates are the main focus in this diet plans.

However, you can't neglect other nutrients. Vegetables are also extremely important, together with a strong serving of protein. From this plans you would have a better idea.

Plan 1

- 0700 Hours: Meal 1 - Oatmeal With Banana Slices/Poached Eggs
- 0900 Hours: Meal 2 - Protein Shake
- 1200 Hours: Meal 3 - Skinless Chicken Breast With Olive Oil + Brown Rice + Broccoli (Steamed)
- 1600 Hours: Meal 4 - Green Beans
- 1900 Hours: Meal 5 - Salmon Fillet + Sweet Potato

Plan 2

- 0700 Hours: Meal 1 - Egg White Pancakes + Fruits Salad
- 0900 Hours: Meal 2 - Yogurt + Fruit
- 1200 Hours: Meal 3 - Vegetable Curry + Brown Rice
- 1600 Hours: Meal 4: Fruit Salad With Greens And Chicken
- 1900 Hours: Meal 5: Chilli With Turkey, Kidney Beans And Salsa + Steamed Vegetables

As you can see from both the meals, there is a balance of carbohydrates, vegetables and protein. These three are the main nutrient you need.

I also recommend drinking milk at the end of the day to give you extra protein.

Remember that these meal plans are to just give you an idea. Create your own ones. You can search for ideas from the internet.

Key Pointers

When you are eating for metabolism, there are some things which you need to bear in mind. These are things that many people forget.

Among them include:

1. **Supplements Cannot Boost Your Metabolism.** Anyone who look to build metabolism by eating supplements need to know that boosting metabolism is not just about losing weight. You are wasting your money. No research has been done to relate taking supplements with boosting metabolism.

2. **You Can't Take Too Much Of Some Food.** Food like spicy ones and green tea should only be taken on a

moderate level. These are food that are used to be added to other high protein food like meat or tuna. You can't solely depend on such food.

3. **Forget The Diet Pills.** Diet Pills are only for those who want to lose weight. Diet pills would help you burn fat and control your appetite but they don't boost metabolism AT ALL. Besides, taking diet pills is dangerous because you would most probably be dependent on them on the long term. You will need to take more of it to get the same effect as before. If you insist on taking them, make sure you read the box properly first. Most pills of such nature have serious consequences. An even better way is to consult your doctor.

Keep in mind of all these advice when deciding to put anything into your mouth.

I have covered on exercising and eating. In the next chapter, I would deal with the final and perhaps most important part of boosting metabolism: How to handle stress.

How To De-Stress Yourself

Stress is commonly accepted to be an ordinary part of life. This section of this book is for you to understand stress and manage it.

One important thing that I need to explain is the fact that stress isn't a part of life. We, as a society, has accepted stress as a part of life to a point that we allow our lives to be stressful. Yes, we live in a fast-paced culture driven by urgency and deadlines.

But, you don't have to be stressed when you deal with them.

People around us are living in this belief that if they get more things done in a shorter amount of time, they are better. Everything from work, relationships to family becomes a great balancing act. Tension, anxiety and fear become very common.

Add to that, emotional problems like death of loved ones and divorce become extra pressure for your life.

Stress, therefore, becomes an important part of boosting your metabolism because it could seriously affect your metabolism over the long term. Your health would be affected.

Link Between Stress And Metabolism

In our body, there is a hormone called as cortisol. Cortisol aids in several body functions. It helps the release of insulin for blood sugar stability; regulate blood pressure, increase immunity and metabolism of glucose.

Cortisol, in small increases could be extremely beneficial as it results in quick and healthy jolt of energy and immunity. It also gives you a higher pain threshold and better memory.

However, all is not positive. If cortisol is released too much or too often, it results in:

- Imbalance Blood Sugar
- Blood Pressure Gets Highers
- Lower Cognitive Ability
- Decreased Immunity
- Decrease In Muscle Tissue And Bone Density

Cortisol also aims the stimulation of amino acid released from your muscles to be converted to glucose. It would serve as a great energy source for your body to cope with stress.

However, stress is also harmful to the body. It would lead to the production of more acid than what the body needs. Our bodies have a balance between 80% alkaline and 20% acid. If you have too much acid, you would decrease your immunity and make you extremely vulnerable to sickness. And you guessed it, too much acid also affects your metabolism.

To keep your cortisol levels healthy, you need to effectively cope with stress. Once your body goes into stress, you need to learn how to relax yourself.

Methods Of De-Stressing

There are numerous methods to de-stress yourself. Since there are many reasons of stress, you need to decide for yourself what works for you.

How To Recharge Yourself Quickly

1) **Massage** - This is my personal favorite. Also known as touch therapy, massaging is extremely beneficial in loosening up your joints and muscles. When we are stressed, they may be tensed up. This is especially so for your back muscles. Massage could also be combined with aromatherapy.

2) **Aromatherapy** - This method is a great way to release stress from events that happened throughout the day. The most commonly use oils include lavender and mint. Take a few drops and mix it with water on your oil burner. Combined with meditation, you would find that it is an extremely relaxing. You can even use some aromatherapy when you are tired throughout the day. A five

minute aromatherapy session would do a great way to changing the way your day goes.

3) **Visualization** - Visualization is one of the most effective methods towards reducing stress. You can imagine yourself sitting in a boat with a quiet surroundings. Imagine that the blue sky is in perfect balance as you feel the wind. After some time, you would feel extremely relaxed while you glide around in the boat. There are various visualization technique for relaxation. It is something that requires a lot of creativity.

4) **Music Therapy** - Play some gentle, relaxing music on your player. Sit comfortably on a position, close your eyes and feel the enjoyment of the music washing away the stress. It would

gently wash away your fears and anxieties. Head over to YouTube and search for soothing music from nature like raining sounds and ocean waves.

How To Release Stress For The Long Term

1) **Be Positive** - There has been increasing research on how positive thinking greatly affects a person health and well-being. According to research, having positive thoughts make your physical healthy better. Bad thoughts react negatively and good thoughts react positively. Therefore always have pleasant thoughts.

In any situation, try to find for a positive way to looking at things. If you have something to look forward to, always try to visualize the positive outcome of thinks. Imagine how you can have the best career, relationship and friendship. Feel the feelings of those positive feelings.

2) **Release Negative Feelings And Thoughts** - When you indulge in negative feelings and thoughts, it is similar to maintaining acid in your body. It is no wonder than tension and fear eventually lead to heartburn or indigestion. Resentment meanwhile would make you more susceptible to high blood pressure.

However, you should never suppress your feelings. Always look for way to express your negative feelings. Doing so would lead to higher acid levels. You need to feel the feelings that you have, express it well and gently let go.

3) **Take Up Yoga** - Yoga is one of the most incredible ways to release stress. Besides, yoga can fire up your metabolism. Yoga has many different postures which assists your organs by strengthening them for metabolism.

To release you from stress, one of the highly recommended position is the corpse pose. As the name mentions, you just need to lie down like a corpse.

4) **Daily Meditation** - Making meditation a daily habit is one of the best habits you could have.

Meditation brings you a peace of mind and trains you to be better able to cope with stress. Meditation doesn't have to be complex. You just need to sit down on a cross-legged position and focus on your breathe. Focus on your entire body and feel the gentle release of tension from your body.

Once you feel relaxed, you can sit still while letting thoughts come into your mind. Observe the thoughts that you have in your mind and detach yourself from them. This is so you don't mindlessly attach yourself to any thoughts that may bring you stress in your thoughts. Just naturally allow any thoughts to enter your mind and then let it leave your mind.

5) **Always Plan Ahead In Your Life** - If you feel that your stressful moments is always recurring, you should always plan ahead. Once you have identified the reasons for your stress, see if you could avoid it.

If, for example, one of the reasons for your stress is because of the traffic that you face in the morning, you should spent time planning to go out earlier than normal to avoid the traffic.

These simple things go a great way to ensuring that you can manage your stress better.

Moreover, if you find yourself being stressed when you work for long hours, you will need to modify how and what you eat. You still need to understand the principles of fast metabolism diet and follow them religiously.

To manage stress well, you would especially need Vitamin C as it helps your body cope better with stress. Eat more citrus fruits and strawberries. Other than that, your diet remains pretty much the same - focusing on carbohydrates, vegetables and protein.

Importance Of Sleep

While you are asleep, your body takes the time to fully recover from your rigorous exercises. This is also a very important time for your muscles to grow. Your muscles don't grow while you work out; they grow while you are asleep. If you don't sleep well, your muscles won't grow well regardless of how much effort you put in your workout.

When you lack sleep, you also prevent your body from being in top condition for your workouts. Having insufficient energy means that you can't push yourself. You would find yourself being tired very quickly and the quality of your workout diminishing.

Research has also shown that if you lack sleep, you won't be able to process your carbohydrates well. The glucose you take also would not be properly metabolized and this results in increased hunger and decreased metabolism in the long run.

Make sure that you get at least eight hours of quality sleep each night. This helps the body properly recharge for your next day's work out. The best period for sleep is from 10pm to 6am. Try sticking to this schedule. Sleeping early ensures that you would be able to get all the benefits from resting.

Key Points

For many people I know, de-stressing is perhaps the toughest part of this three part course. This is because most people are so used to their own habits that changing them would take a lot of time and effort.

Most people has incorporate stress into their daily lives without realizing. To reverse that, you should learn to take things slowly. Try to clear up your daily schedule and find some quiet time alone each day. Just a few minutes a day would go a long way towards slowing down the pace of your workday.

To me, the best habit that I can recommend you is daily meditation. You don't have to sit in meditation for an hour a day. Just a mere five or ten minute would do wonders for your everyday stress reduction.

There has been numerous studies that show that meditators are less stressed and are better equipped to deal with the changes in everyday life. If you feel that your schedule is tough and you can't avoid staying up late, take more time to sleep on the weekends.

A lack of sleep causes many problems from cognitive impairment to a lack of energy. Your body wouldn't function as well as they should and would affect your metabolism as well.

Always plan time to de-stress. It will boost your metabolism in a long term.

Chapter Five: Take Action Now

Knowing is important. But taking action is even more important. From the previous chapter, you have learned the importance of exercising, eating and de-stressing.

These three components are important for the boosting of your mechanism. Metabolism is the process of converting calories into energy for storage and immediate use. Without a doubt, metabolism is perhaps one of the body's most important function. It works every second of your life.

As you now know the basics of metabolism, I have created a summary for you to take action.

1) How To Exercise Smart

- Strength And Resistance Exercises - Build your muscles through these exercises by using a combination of exercises with and without weights. Focus on exercises which work several muscles at once.

- Interval Training - Cardio exercises helps you burn calories. Alternate high and moderate intensity exercises.

- Alternate Exercises - Alternate strength training with interval training. Have one day of total rest for your muscles to recover.

2) How To Eat Well

- More Is Good - We are focusing on boosting metabolism, not losing weight. Eat more.

- Focus On Carbohydrates And Proteins - These are what drives your metabolism.

- Don't Forget Other Nutrients - Vegetables (Fiber), Calcium And Healthy Fats Shouldn't Be Neglected.

- Eat Breakfast - Breakfast kicks off your metabolism.

- Five To Six Meals A Day - Every two to three hours, take a meal. Small meals count as well. Make it convenient for you to have those meals.

- Eight Hours Of Water A Day.

- Eat One Hour After Every Workout

3) How To De-Stress Yourself

- Recharge Yourself - Through different methods, you can learn to recharge yourself each day.

- Take A Long Term View - By yoga, meditation and positive thinking; you would be able to better handle your stressful situations.

This summary would do yourself a great deal towards boosting your metabolism. Remember, that knowing is not enough. You must also do.

This plan is 'foolproof'. The only thing that you need to worry about is all the excuses that you would give yourself. You need to stop making excuses and start taking action once and for all if you want a different life.

When you feel demotivated, take time to go through the visualization that I recommended at the beginning of this book. The results would be astounding.

Good luck and all the best in having a healthier and better life for yourself.

Resources

Want to cook more delicious food to ensure that you would be able to keep up with the metabolic diet. The link below would show you how to cook amazing metabolic diets that would help you achieve your goal of boosting metabolism.

http://metabolicchef.wellbeingvalley.com

Want to not only build metabolism but muscles as well? Check the link below...

http://metabolictraining.wellbeingvalley.com

www.ingramcontent.com/pod-product-compliance
Lightning Source LLC
Chambersburg PA
CBHW070553290526
45790CB00002B/672